Adel ElHennawy

First-Time Mom's Ultimate Pregnancy Companion

Your Hassle-Free Guide to a Healthy Pregnancy, Positive Birth, and Thriving Baby, Risk-Free, in 20 Minutes a Day

This book was professionally typeset on Reedsy
Find out more at reedsy.com

Contents

1.

2.

3.

4.

5.

6.

7.

8.

9.

10.

11.

1

Introduction

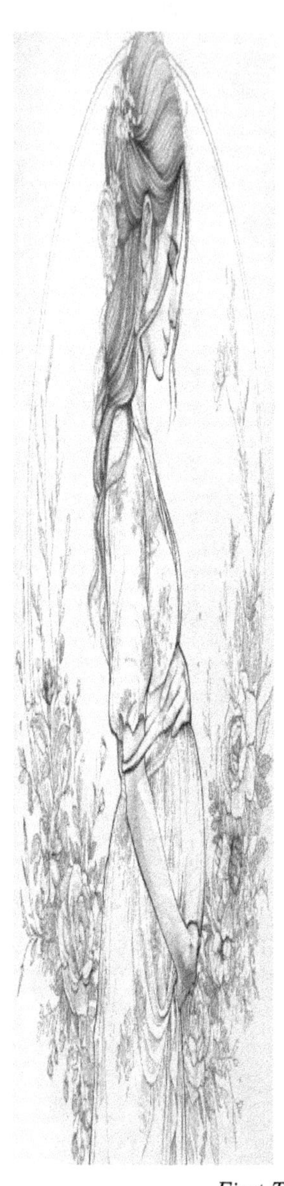

First-Time Mom's Ultimate Companion

"First-Time Mom's Ultimate Pregnancy Companion" is your guide for navigating pregnancy, birth, and the initial parenting phase. It offers a 20-minute daily routine focusing on essential pregnancy and newborn care, designed for the modern, busy expectant mom. This routine is crafted to easily integrate into any part of your day, ensuring you get necessary health maintenance and birth preparation tips.

The book combines experiences from other moms, expert advice, and the latest prenatal and postnatal care insights. It aims to connect with readers personally, offering motivation and community while addressing common challenges. Topics covered include trimester expectations, birth prep, nutrition, exercise, breastfeeding, postpartum recovery, and life with a newborn.

Topics covered include trimester-by-trimester expectations, birth preparation, nutrition, exercise, breastfeeding, postpartum recovery, and adapting to life with a new baby. The aim is to equip you with the knowledge to make informed decisions for you and your baby's well being, boosting your confidence as you embark on motherhood.

Every pregnancy and parenting journey is unique, but access to trustworthy information and support is crucial. This book seeks to be a comprehensive source of practical advice and support as you navigate the complexities of becoming a parent.

This guide's goal is to empower you with knowledge for making informed decisions, boosting confidence as you enter motherhood, but having trusted information can significantly help. By starting with this guide, you're on your way to a well-informed, confident, and joyful experience of pregnancy and early parenthood.

2

Understanding Your Pregnancy

Main **Idea:** In this chapter, we've taken a practical and informative approach to demystify the pregnancy process. By breaking down what to expect in each trimester and emphasizing essential prenatal care, we aim to equip you with the knowledge and tools needed for a healthy pregnancy journey. This chapter combines straightforward advice with actionable tips, ensuring you feel supported and informed at every stage of your pregnancy.

The First Trimester: What to expect

Embarking on the journey of pregnancy, especially for the first time, is a blend of excitement, anticipation, and, naturally, a myriad of questions about the changes your body will undergo. This subsection aims to be your guide through the initial stage of pregnancy, providing clarity on the early signs, the physical and emotional transformations you might experience, and practical advice on managing common first-trimester symptoms.

- **Physical and Emotional Changes:** The first trimester marks the beginning of significant changes. Physically, you might experience nausea, fatigue, breast tenderness, and frequent urination. Emotionally, fluctuations in hormone levels can lead to mood swings. These symptoms vary in intensity from person to person.

- **Prenatal Care:** Your initial prenatal visit is crucial. It typically involves a comprehensive health check, including blood tests for genetic and health conditions, urine tests for infections, and possibly your first ultrasound. This visit is an opportunity to discuss your health history, current medications, and any lifestyle changes that pregnancy necessitates.

- **Lifestyle Adjustments:** Start taking prenatal vitamins, if you haven't already, focusing on folic acid, iron, and calcium. Moderate exercise, such as walking or prenatal yoga, can help manage fatigue and support physical well-being. Stay hydrated and eat a balanced diet to support your baby's development.

Navigating the Second Trimester: Body Changes and Baby's Growth

The second trimester is often greeted with a sigh of relief by many pregnant women, as it marks a period of decreased nausea and a noticeable increase in energy levels. This subsection is designed to guide you through the significant changes happening in your body and to your growing baby, aiming to prepare you for the adjustments in your lifestyle that these changes necessitate.

Physical Changes: As morning sickness subsides, you may notice an increase in energy. This trimester is when you'll start to show, and you may begin to feel your baby's movements. Back pain and leg cramps can occur as your body adjusts to its growing size.

Ultrasound and Gender Discovery: The anatomy scan, a detailed ultrasound, usually happens between 18 to 22 weeks. It assesses the baby's growth, development, organ function and can often reveal the sex of the baby, if you choose to know. It's a profound opportunity to connect with your baby, seeing them move and even catching glimpses of their personality in utero. Your baby's bones are starting to harden, and they're making movements you might start to feel as gentle flutters at first. These movements will become more pronounced as your baby grows

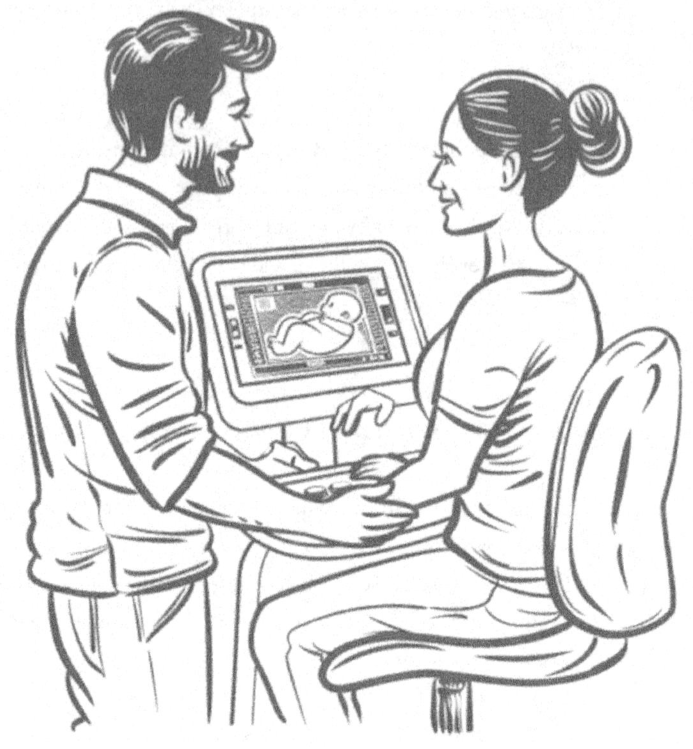

Your First Fetal Ultrasound

Nutrition and Exercise: Your appetite might increase. Focus on nutrient-rich foods that provide the energy and vitamins that support both your health and your baby's development. Continuing with regular, moderate gentle exercises and stretches, particularly those focusing on your back and pelvic floor, can offer relief and strengthen your body for the coming months, adjusting as necessary to remain comfortable and safe. It's also a time when many women report feeling their best during pregnancy, making it an excellent time to engage in prenatal yoga or water aerobics, which can help maintain your fitness and boost your mood, without putting too much strain on your body.

Sleep may start to become more challenging as finding a comfortable position becomes harder. Investing in a good quality pregnancy pillow and adapting a bedtime routine that promotes relaxation can significantly improve your sleep quality.

Adapting your lifestyle during the second trimester to accommodate these changes involves a balanced approach to diet, exercise, and rest. Embracing this period of growth and development, while making necessary adjustments to your daily routine, can help ensure both you and your baby are as healthy and comfortable as possible. This is a time of preparation, connection, and anticipation as you move closer to meeting your baby.

Preparing for the Third Trimester: Final Preparation

Entering the third trimester signifies the final stretch of your pregnancy journey, a time when your body and baby make their last preparations for birth. This subsection aims to inform you about the changes and developments you can expect during this period, offering practical advice to navigate them with ease and confidence.

The third trimester is crucial, focusing on final birth preparations and adjusting to significant body changes. Expect Braxton Hicks contractions as practice for labor. Regular baby movement monitoring is essential; any changes should prompt a consultation with your healthcare provider. Embrace nesting by organizing your home for the baby, but delegate to avoid strain.

Birth Plan

Detail your birth preferences, including pain management and delivery environment wishes, who you want present during delivery, and any specific practices you'd like to follow, such as immediate skin-to-skin contact with your baby in a birth plan. Discuss this with your healthcare team to align expectations.

Choosing a Pediatrician

Select a pediatrician that matches your parenting style. Schedule a meeting to ensure they're a good fit and address any concerns.

Hospital Bag

Pack essentials for your hospital stay, including comfortable clothing for you and the baby, toiletries, and important documents. Include items for your support person.

Managing Discomfort

Incorporate gentle exercises to ease third-trimester discomfort. Practice relaxation techniques and find comfortable sleeping positions to maximize rest.

Essential Prenatal Nutrition and Exercise

Navigating the nutritional needs and exercise routines during pregnancy is crucial for the health of both the mother and the developing baby. This subsection aims to demystify prenatal nutrition by highlighting the key nutrients required and offering strategies for incorporating them into your daily diet. Additionally, we'll explore safe and effective exercise routines that support your body's changing needs throughout each trimester of pregnancy.

Nutrition Needs

Focus on critical nutrients: Essential nutrients include folic acid, vital for preventing neural tube defects; iron, to increase blood volume and prevent anemia; calcium, for developing your baby's bones and teeth; and DHA, an omega-3 fatty acid important for brain development. Include diverse food sources like leafy green vegetables for folic acid, lean meats and legumes for iron, dairy products or fortified plant milks for calcium, and fatty fish or algae-based supplements for DHA. Use smoothies for an easy nutrient intake and balance cravings with healthy choices.

Exercise Guidelines

Exercise during pregnancy not only helps maintain fitness but also prepares your body for childbirth. It can reduce pregnancy-related discomforts like back pain, improve sleep, and increase stamina needed for labor and delivery. Maintain fitness with walking, swimming, prenatal yoga, and adapted strength training. Prioritize pelvic floor strengthening and flexibility. Adjust activities by trimester: moderate exercise in the first like walking or swimming to help manage fatigue and nausea, incorporate more structured exercise routines and activity in the second, and birth-preparation exercises that maintain flexibility and strengthen the muscles you'll use during labor, such as squats and pelvic tilts in the third.

Consult your healthcare provider to customize nutrition and exercise plans to your pregnancy needs.

3

Preparing for Birth

Main Idea: In this chapter, we aim to provide comprehensive guidance on preparing for birth, covering everything from creating a detailed birth plan to understanding the stages of labor and exploring pain relief options. By equipping you with this knowledge, our goal is to empower you to approach childbirth with confidence, making informed decisions for a positive birth experience.

Creating Your Birth Plan: Options and Considerations

Purpose of a Birth Plan:

A birth plan is a document communicating your preferences for labor and delivery to your healthcare team. A well-thought-out birth plan covers various aspects of the birthing process, including the type of environment you envision—be it a hospital, birthing center, or a home birth. Specify the ambiance you'd prefer; some women request dim lighting, soft music, or the presence of personal items to create a calming environment.

Pain management is another critical area; detail your preferences for natural pain relief methods such as breathing techniques, hydrotherapy, or the use of a birthing ball, as well as your stance on medical interventions like epidurals or other forms of analgesia. Evaluate the benefits and considerations of each, discussing with your healthcare provider to align with your birth plan. Consider the role of support persons.

The role of birthing assistants, such as Doulas, can also be included in your plan. Doulas provide emotional and physical support throughout labor and delivery, which can be invaluable in navigating the birthing process. and your views on medical interventions. Additionally, consider how you feel about various medical procedures, such as episiotomies, the use of forceps or vacuums, and under what circumstances you would be open to a cesarean section.

It's important to research and understand these procedures ahead of time, so you can make informed decisions.

- Discuss flexibility with your healthcare provider, as labor and delivery can be unpredictable, and situations may arise that require deviating from your plan to ensure the safety and health of you and your baby.

Understanding Labor: Understanding Labor: Signs, Stages, and When to Go to the Hospital

- Labor is a profoundly personal and varied experience for each woman, characterized by several stages that mark the progression towards giving birth. Labor is generally categorized into three main stages: early labor, active labor, and the delivery of the placenta.
- **Early Labor:** This first phase is often the longest but usually the least intense. Signs include irregular contractions, experience the breaking of your waters (rupture of membranes) and a bloody show, which is a small amount of blood-tinged mucus indicating the cervix is beginning to dilate. During early labor, you might find it helpful to stay relaxed, hydrated, and nourished, and to keep monitoring the frequency and intensity of your contractions.
- **Active Labor:** Your contractions will become more regular, longer, stronger, and closer together, typically about 3-5 minutes apart. This is when your cervix dilates from about 6 cm to 10 cm. Pain and discomfort become more pronounced. This is the time to head to the hospital or birthing center. Effective coping strategies include focused breathing, massage, warm baths or showers, and the support of your birthing team.
- **Transition:** Often considered the most challenging part of labor, the transition phase occurs as the cervix completes dilation to 10 cm.

Contractions are very strong, with little to no rest in between. Though intense, this phase is usually brief compared to the others.

- **Delivery of the Baby:** The moment has arrived to push and bring your baby into the world. You'll rely heavily on your healthcare provider's guidance during this stage, utilizing your energy to push effectively during contractions.

- **Delivery of the Placenta:** After your baby is born, you'll deliver the placenta, marking the final stage of labor. This usually happens within 5 to 30 minutes post-delivery, with mild contractions that are less intense than those for birthing the baby.

- **Recognizing the signs of true labor versus false labor, known as Braxton Hicks contractions, is crucial:** True labor contractions progressively become more regular, stronger, and closer together, while Braxton Hicks are usually irregular and do not increase in intensity.

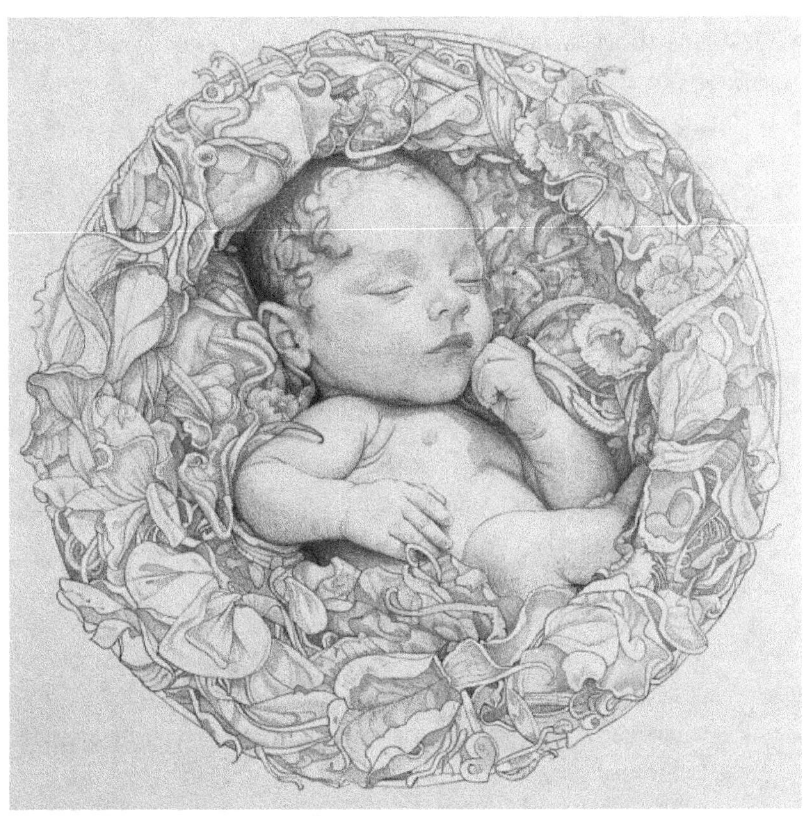

Delivery Of Your Baby

- **Pain Relief Options: From Natural Methods to Medical Interventions**

Labor and delivery can be intensely painful for many women, and how you choose to manage this pain is a personal decision that should align with your birth plan and preferences.

Natural Pain Relief Methods: For those interested in a medication-free birth experience, several natural pain relief techniques can be effective. These include:

- **Breathing Exercises**
- **Meditation and Visualization**
- **Movement and Position Changes**
- **Water Birth**
- **Massage and Acupressure**

Medical Interventions: When natural methods are not enough, or if you prefer more direct forms of pain relief, several medical options are available:

- **Epidurals:** One of the most common pain relief methods during labor, an epidural involves administering pain medication through a catheter in the lower back.
- **Spinal Blocks:** Similar to epidurals but typically used for quick pain relief during later stages of labor or for cesarean deliveries.
- **Analgesics:** These medications can reduce pain without causing a loss of sensation or muscle movement. They can be administered intravenously or through injections but may affect both mother and baby to some degree.

Benefits and Considerations:

Natural techniques: can offer a sense of control and minimal intervention but may not provide complete pain relief for all.

Medical interventions: while effective at managing pain, can have side effects and may impact the labor process or your mobility.

Making a decision about pain relief during labor involves weighing the pros and cons of each method, considering your pain tolerance, and discussing options with your healthcare provider.

What to Pack: Your Hospital Bag Checklist

Packing your hospital bag is a key step in your final preparations for childbirth. Comprehensive checklist of essentials for you and your baby, ensuring a comfortable and stress-free hospital stay.

For the Mother:

- **Comfortable Clothing:** including a robe or nightgown that is breastfeeding accessible if you plan to nurse.
- **Toiletries:** toothbrush, toothpaste, hairbrush, deodorant, face wash, lip balm and any other personal care items you use daily.
- **Important Documents:** Bring any necessary paperwork, including your ID, insurance information, and your birth plan.
- **Snacks and Drinks:** Pack your favorite non-perishable snacks and drinks to keep you energized and hydrated. Hospitals do provide meals.
- **Entertainment and Relaxation Items:** Include items such as books, magazines, a tablet, or a music player with headphones to help you relax during early labor.
- **Going Home Outfit:** Choose something comfortable to wear at home. So maternity clothes are often still the most comfortable option.

For the Baby:

- **Outfits:** Pack a few different sizes of newborn clothes including socks or booties and a hat, as babies need help staying warm.
- **Blankets:** Bring a couple of soft, warm blankets for swaddling your baby in the hospital and for the ride home.
- **Car Seat:** Though not something you'll pack in your bag, ensure you have a properly installed car seat to safely transport your baby home.
- **Diapers and Wipes:** The hospital typically provides newborn diapers and sensitive wipes for your baby's delicate skin.

Additional Tips:

- **Pack Early:** Aim to have your bag packed by the 36th week of pregnancy, as labor can sometimes come earlier than expected.

- **Separate Bags:** Consider packing separate bags for labor and postpartum.

Check Hospital Policies: Some hospitals provide certain supplies, so check ahead to avoid unnecessary packing.

4

The First Weeks at Home

Main Idea: Throughout this chapter, the focus is on providing you with the knowledge and tools needed to navigate the first weeks at home with confidence and compassion. By understanding the fundamentals of postpartum recovery, newborn care, bonding, and overcoming challenges, you'll be better equipped to enjoy and thrive during this special time with your new baby.

Postpartum Recovery: Physical and Emotional Health

The journey through postpartum recovery is a deeply personal experience that encompasses both physical healing and emotional adjustment.

Physical Recovery

You may experience a variety of symptoms in the weeks following delivery, including but not limited to, soreness, fatigue, and changes in hormonal levels that can impact your overall physical well-being

- **Rest:** Prioritize sleep to aid healing. Try to sleep when your baby sleeps.
- **Nutrition:** Eat a balanced diet rich in vitamins, minerals, and protein to support tissue repair and maintain energy.
- **Gentle Exercise:** Start with light activities like walking. Consider postpartum yoga but listen to your body and avoid overexertion.

Emotional Well-being

The postpartum period can indeed be a roller coaster, with highs of joy and love for your new baby, interspersed with moments of exhaustion, frustration, and potential feelings of sadness or anxiety

- **Emotional Fluctuations:** It's normal to feel joy, exhaustion, and even sadness. Acknowledge these feelings without judgment.
- **Support Network:** Lean on family, friends, and professionals for support and practical help.
- **Self-care:** Allocate time for activities you enjoy and relax. Self-care is crucial for emotional recovery.

Recognizing More Serious Conditions

- Be aware of postpartum depression (PPD) and anxiety symptoms, such as prolonged sadness, apathy, feelings of worthlessness or excessive worry. If these feelings persist, seek professional help promptly.

Basics of Newborn Care: Feeding, Sleeping, and Diapering

- Caring for a newborn brings a mix of immense joy and significant responsibility, requiring new parents to quickly learn the essentials on the foundational aspects of newborn care. This section delivers direct guidance on essential newborn care areas—feeding, sleeping, and diapering—to help new parents manage with confidence.

Feeding Basics

- **Recognize Hunger Cues:** Look for signs like rooting and fussiness.
- **Breastfeeding:** Focus on comfortable positioning and ensuring a proper latch for success.
- **Formula Feeding:** Select an appropriate formula, prepare bottles correctly, and stick to a feeding schedule.
- **Feeding Frequency:** Feed on demand to accommodate growth spurts, tracking feeding times and baby's weight.

Sleep Strategies

- **Safe Sleep Environment:** Place your baby on their back in a crib or bassinet without soft bedding or toys.
- **Sleep Patterns:** Expect 14-17 hours of sleep per day in short intervals.
- **Bedtime Routine:** Start a simple routine to signal sleep time, but anticipate nighttime awakenings for feedings.

Diapering

- **Preparation:** Have a stock of diapers and wipes and a comfortable changing area.
- **Frequency:** Change diapers around 10 times daily, monitoring fit and skin condition to avoid rash.
- **Health Checks:** Use diaper changes to assess hydration and health through urine and stool appearance.

By focusing on these key aspects, new parents can effectively address their newborn's basic needs, ensuring proper care and comfort in the crucial first week at home.

Bonding with Your Baby: Establishing Connection

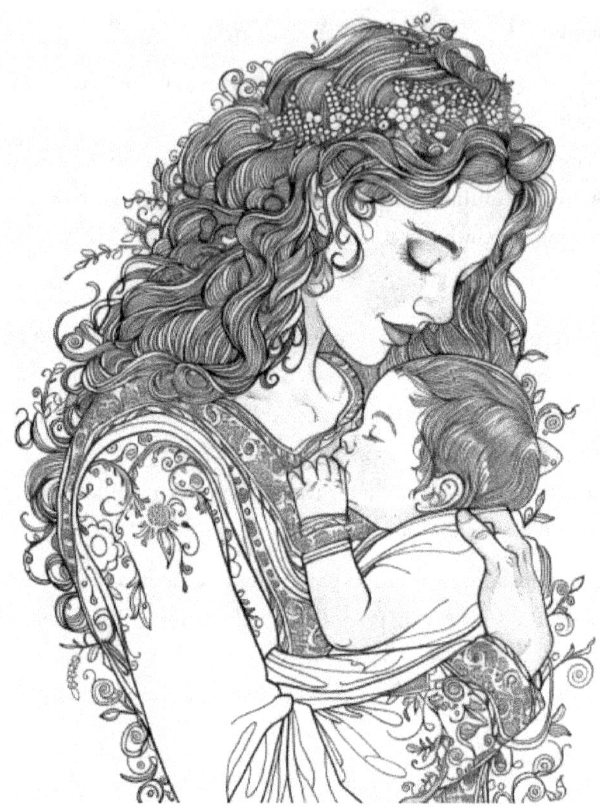

Bonding With Your Baby

Bonding is essential for your baby's emotional development and strengthening your relationship. This section offers strategies to enhance bonding, emphasizing the importance of early, attentive interactions.

Skin-to-Skin Contact

- **Importance:** Provides warmth, comfort, and security, promoting breastfeeding success and stabilizing baby's vital signs.
- **Practice:** Hold your baby against your skin regularly to foster a strong emotional connection. Skin-to-skin contact can also facilitate breastfeeding success

Responsive Feeding

- **Approach:** Pay attention to hunger cues and feed your baby in a way that promotes closeness, whether breastfeeding or bottle-feeding.
- **Benefit:** Builds trust by meeting nutritional needs and offering comfort.

Gentle Play

- **Activities:** Talk, make eye contact, sing, and play with your baby's limbs gently.
- **Outcome:** Stimulates development and creates joyful moments of connection.

Reading Babies Cues

- **Skill:** Learn to recognize and respond to your baby's signals for hunger, comfort, or sleep.
- **Impact:** Establishes a responsive care pattern, forming the basis of secure attachment.

Consistent Care

- **Strategy:** Maintain regular caregiving routines and responses.
- **Result:** Reinforces your baby's sense of security and strengthens your bond.

By incorporating these bonding strategies, you're setting a strong foundation for your baby's emotional well-being and your enduring relationship. Bonding is a rewarding process that assures your baby of love and security, crucial for their optimal start in life.

Navigating Challenges: Colic, Sleep Issues, and Feeding Difficulties

The initial weeks with your newborn might bring challenges like colic, disrupted sleep, and feeding issues. This section outlines practical advice to manage these common problems effectively.

Colic Management

- **Symptoms:** Intense crying in a healthy baby, typically in the late afternoon or evening.
- **Soothing Strategies:** Try rocking, swaddling, white noise, or gentle walks. Always check for basic needs like hunger or a diaper change first.
- **Support:** Consult your pediatrician for advice. Remember, colic is temporary, and support groups can offer coping strategies.

Sleep Issues

- **Newborn Sleep:** Expect irregular sleep patterns with frequent nighttime awakenings.
- **Bedtime Routine:** Introduce a calming routine, including baths, massages, or soft music, to help signal sleep time.
- **Environment:** Ensure the sleeping area is safe, quiet, and comfortable.
- **Patience and Consistency:** Regular routines and a safe sleep environment gradually improve sleep patterns.

Feeding Difficulties

- **Common Problems:** Issues may arise with latching, milk supply, or formula tolerance.
- **Breastfeeding Support:** A lactation consultant can offer tailored advice and solutions for breastfeeding challenges.
- **Bottle-feeding Tips:** Experiment with different bottles and nipples to find what works best for your baby.
- **Relaxed Feeding:** Observe hunger cues and create a calm feeding environment to help reduce difficulties.

Seeking Help

- It's important to seek assistance from healthcare professionals, parenting groups, or your support network when facing these challenges. Getting help is a sign of proactive parenting, not a weakness.

By applying these strategies and utilizing available resources, you can navigate the early parenting challenges with greater ease, ensuring both you and your baby have a more comfortable adjustment period.

5

Feeding Your Baby

- **Main Idea:** This chapter aims to empower you with the knowledge and skills needed to navigate the feeding process, from the earliest days of your baby's life through to their first taste of solid food and beyond. By understanding the basics of breastfeeding, bottle-feeding, introducing solids, and meeting your baby's nutritional needs, you'll be well-equipped to provide your baby with the best possible start in their nutritional journey

Breastfeeding Basics: Techniques, Tips, and Troubleshooting

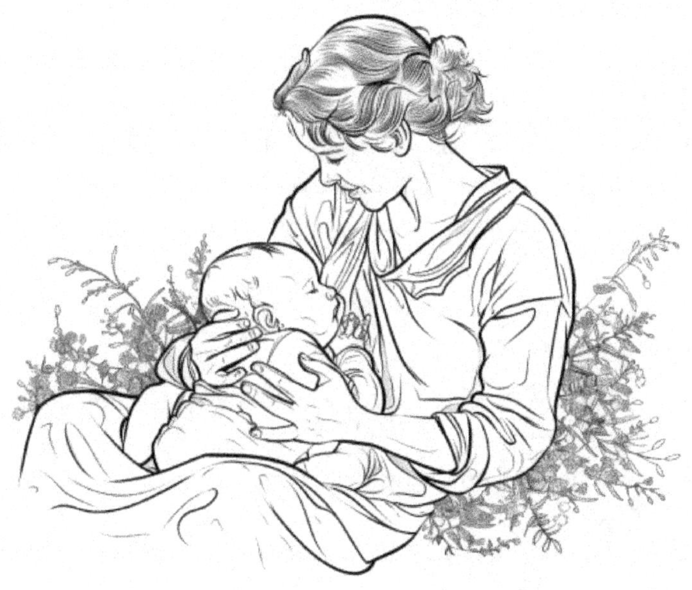

Breastfeeding, while a natural process, often requires patience and practice to master. This subsection is designed to guide new mothers through the early stages of breastfeeding, offering essential techniques, helpful tips, and solutions to common breastfeeding challenges, offers guidance on mastering breastfeeding, from establishing a good latch to managing milk supply to ensure a successful and fulfilling breastfeeding experience.

Achieving the Right Latch

- **Importance:** Essential for effective breastfeeding; involves more than just the nipple, including a good portion of the areola.
- **Signs of a Good Latch:** Baby's mouth wide, chin and nose touching the breast, and visible swallowing.
- **Adjustment:** If the latch causes pain or is shallow, break suction gently and retry for a better latch.

Comfortable Breastfeeding Positions

- **Variety:** Try different positions—cradle, cross-cradle, football hold, side-lying—to find what's comfortable.
- **Benefits:** Changing positions helps prevent soreness and ensures effective milk removal.

Maintaining Milk Supply

- **Frequency:** Breastfeed on demand, about every 2-3 hours or 8-12 times per 24 hours.
- **Indicators:** Look for early hunger signs like rooting or sucking on fingers.
- **Support:** Drink fluids, eat well, and rest to aid milk production.

Addressing Common Breastfeeding Issues

- **Nipple Soreness:** Normal at first but addresses severe pain. Check latch, use nipple cream or expressed milk for relief.
- **Engorgement:** Breastfeed often, apply warm compresses before and cold compresses after feeds. Hand express or pump if needed.
- **Sufficient Milk Intake:** Look for steady weight gain, sufficient wet/dirty diapers, and baby satisfaction post-feeding. Consult a professional if concerned.

For personalized assistance, lactation consultants and healthcare providers are valuable resources.

Bottle Feeding: Choosing Formula and Bottles

For many parents, Bottle-feeding, whether with formula or expressed breast milk, is a vital part of many parents' feeding routines. This section offers straightforward advice on selecting suitable formula, bottles, and nipples to ensure a positive feeding experience for you and your baby.

Choosing the Right Formula

- **Options:** Formula types include cow's milk-based, soy-based, hypoallergenic, and special dietary needs formulas.
- **Consultation:** Discuss with your pediatrician to choose the best formula type, considering any allergies or sensitivities.
- **Trial and Error:** It may take trying several formulas to find the right match for your baby.

Selecting Bottles and Nipples

- **Materials:** Bottles come in plastic, glass, and silicone. Choose based on preference and practicality.
- **Nipple Varieties:** Nipples differ in shape, flow rate, and material. Select one that suits your baby's sucking strength and mimics natural breastfeeding as closely as possible.
- **Flow Rate:** Ensure the nipple's flow rate is neither too fast nor too slow for your baby's comfort.

Preparation and Storage

- **Formula Preparation:** Follow formula preparation instructions carefully for safety and nutrition.
- **Breast Milk Storage:** Store expressed milk in clean containers, adhering to refrigeration and thawing guidelines.
- **Warming:** Warm bottles to body temperature for comfort, testing milk temperature to avoid scalding.

Making Bottle-Feeding a Bonding Experience

- **Bonding:** Use bottle-feeding times to bond with your baby through close holding, eye contact, and interaction.
- **Switching Arms:** Mimic breastfeeding by switching arms mid-feed to support balanced development.

This guide is designed to simplify bottle-feeding, helping you make informed decisions about formula and feeding equipment. By focusing on your baby's specific needs and maintaining safe feeding practices, bottle-feeding can be a nourishing and bonding experience that supports your baby's development and well-being.

Introducing Solids: When and How

The transition to solid foods marks a pivotal milestone in your baby's growth and development, introducing them to a new world of flavors and textures. This subsection aims to provide clear guidance on recognizing the right time to start solids, understanding your baby's readiness signs, and implementing a successful and enjoyable introduction to solid food.

Timing and Readiness

- **When to Start:** The American Academy of Pediatrics suggests introducing solids around 6 months, aligning with your baby's developmental readiness.
- **Readiness Signs:** Look for sitting up with little support, interest in your food, opening mouth for food, and the ability to swallow food without pushing it out with their tongue.

Methods: Purees vs. Baby-Led Weaning

- **Traditional Weaning:** Starts with smooth purees to easily introduce a variety of nutrients.

- **Baby-Led Weaning:** Offers whole foods for self-feeding, promoting motor skills and self-regulation.
- **Combination:** You may combine both methods to fit your baby's preferences and needs.

Introducing Flavors and Textures

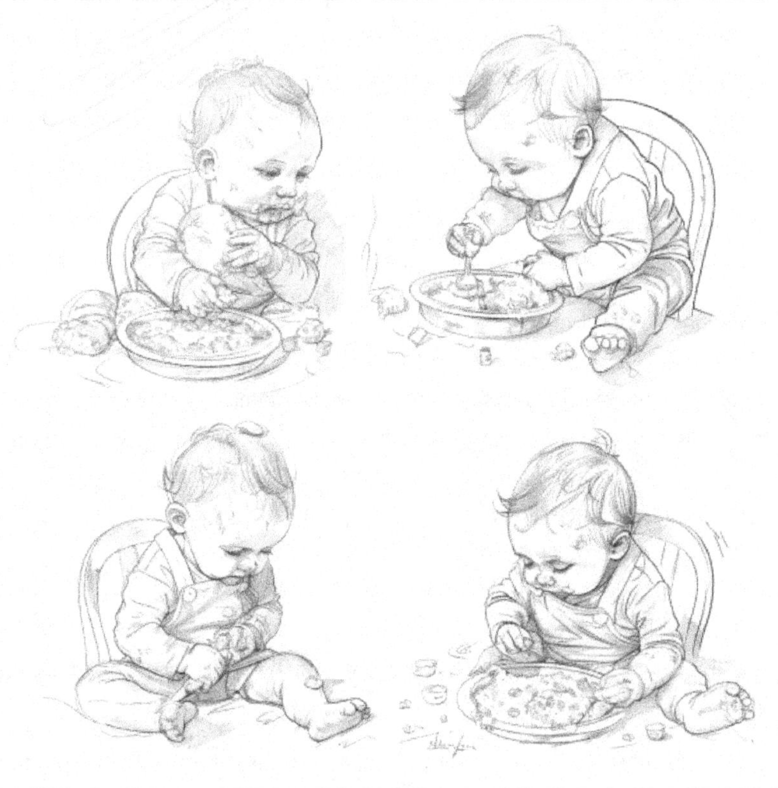

- **Initial Foods:** Begin with single-ingredient purees or soft foods, introducing new items one at a time every few days to check for allergies.

- **Progression:** Gradually increase the variety, including iron-rich foods like fortified cereals or pureed meats, especially important for breastfed babies.
- **Mealtime Environment:** Encourage family meal participation, adapt family foods for baby, and embrace the mess as part of the learning and enjoyment.

Safety and Enjoyment

- **Supervision:** Always watch your baby during meals to prevent choking.
- **Food Preparation:** Start with soft, mashable foods, introducing common allergens one at a time while monitoring for reactions.
- **Positive Environment:** Create stress-free mealtimes, allowing your baby to explore and play with food, fostering a healthy relationship with eating.

Nutritional Needs: Ensuring a Balanced Diet

As your baby grows and develops, their nutritional requirements evolve, necessitating a diet that supports their rapid growth and developmental milestones. This subsection is dedicated to outlining the essential nutrients needed during the first year of life and providing practical advice on how to create a balanced diet that meets these needs.

Essential Nutrients for Babies: During the first year, a baby's diet should include a wide range of nutrients:

- **Proteins:** Support growth with sources like lean meats, beans, tofu, and yogurt.
- **Healthy Fats:** Necessary for brain development, found in avocados, olive oil, and fatty fish.
- **Iron:** Critical for cognitive development, especially for breastfed babies. Include iron-fortified cereals, pureed meats, and leafy greens.

- **Calcium and Vitamin D:** Important for bone health, available in dairy and fortified alternatives.
- **Vitamins A, C, E:** Boost the immune system and skin health. Incorporate carrots, sweet potatoes, citrus fruits, and berries.

Balancing Diet Options

- **Homemade vs. Store-Bought:** Homemade food allows ingredient control, while store-bought offers convenience. Read labels for wholesome ingredients and balance both types for variety.
- **Introducing New Foods:** Gradually introduce new items. Persistence is key; babies may need several exposures to accept new foods. Offer a range of textures and flavors without pressure.

Establishing Healthy Eating Habits

- **Role Modeling:** Demonstrate healthy eating habits, as babies emulate their parents.
- **Encourage Self-Feeding:** Promote independence and help babies learn hunger and fullness cues by encouraging self-feeding at an early age.
- **Positive Mealtime Routines:** Create stress-free mealtimes, continue offering diverse foods, and establish routines that make eating a positive experience.

6

Baby's Health and Development

Main Idea: Ensuring the health and fostering the development of your baby are among the primary concerns for any parent. This chapter is designed to guide you through the essential aspects of monitoring your baby's health, understanding developmental milestones, adhering to vaccination schedules, and addressing common health concerns.

Regular Checkups and Vaccinations:

Regular pediatric checkups and vaccinations are essential for your baby's health, offering protection against numerous preventable diseases. This section outlines a schedule for well-baby visits and recommended vaccinations during the first year, ensuring your baby stays on track with their health milestones.

Initial and Ongoing Checkups

- **Newborn Screening:** Conducted shortly after birth to detect various conditions early.
- **Well-Baby Visits:** Scheduled at 1, 2, 4, 6, 9, and 12 months for growth, development assessments, and vaccinations.

Vaccination Schedule

- **Birth:** Hepatitis B (1st dose), Respiratory Syncytial Virus (RSV-mab [Nirsevimab]) depending on maternal RSV status.
- **1-2 Month:** Hepatitis B (2nd dose).

- **2 Months:** Rotavirus 1st dose, DTaP (Diphtheria, Tetanus, and Pertussis 1st dose), Hib (Haemophilus Influenza type b 1st dose), IPV (Poliovirus Vaccine 1st dose), PCV15, PCV 20 (Pneumococcal Conjugate Vaccine 1st dose), and Rotavirus (1st dose).
- **4 Months:** Rotavirus 2nd dose, DTaP (2nd dose), Hib (2nd dose), IPV (2nd dose), PCV15, PCV 20 (2nd dose), and Rotavirus (2nd dose).
- **6 Months:** DTaP (3rd dose), Hib (3rd dose), IPV (3rd dose; may be given at 6-15 months), PCV15, PCV 20 (3rd dose), Rotavirus (3rd dose), Hepatitis B (3rd dose).
- **6-12 Months:** Seasonal Influenza Vaccine, timed with the flu season.
- **12-15 Months:** Measles, Mumps, Rubella (MMR 1st dose), Varicella (1st dose)

Adhering to this vaccination schedule is critical for protecting your baby against serious illnesses. Vaccinations are most effective when administered according to the recommended timelines, equipping your baby with immunity ahead of potential exposure to diseases.

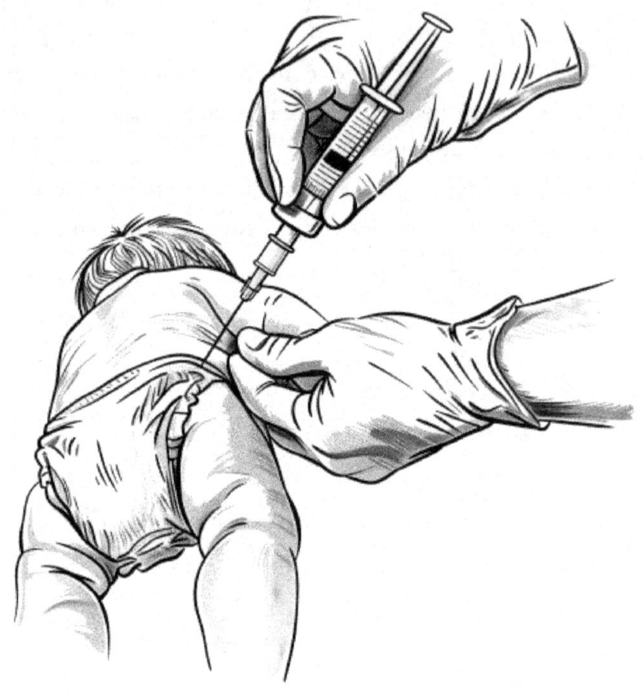

Newborn Vaccination

Importance of Vaccination Records

Keep a detailed record of all vaccinations and present it during pediatric visits. If you have any concerns or questions about vaccinations, discussing them with your pediatrician can offer clarity and help you make informed health decisions for your baby.

Milestones: What to Expect in the First Year

The first year is filled with rapid development in physical, motor, communicative, and social-emotional areas. Here's what to expect from birth to 12 months,providing parents with a comprehensive overview to track their baby's progress and support their burgeoning abilities.

Birth to 3 Months

- **Social and Communication:** Begins to smile socially, coos, and turns head towards sounds.
- **Physical and Motor:** Lifts head during tummy time, showing early motor skill development. Involuntary grasping.

4 to 6 Months

- **Physical Development:** Rolls over both ways, starts to sit with support, and grasps objects voluntarily.
- **Communication:** Babbling sounds, responds to affection, and recognizes names.
- **Social-Emotional:** Shows interest in people and toys, exploring objects by mouth.

7 to 9 Months

- **Mobility:** May crawl, sit without support, and pull to stand with help.
- **Fine Motor Skills:** Uses pincer grasp for small objects.
- **Cognitive and Social:** Responds to simple commands, develops object permanence awareness.

10 to 12 Months

- **Major Milestones:** Stands with assistance, cruises, may take first steps. Begins to use simple gestures and say words like "mama" or "dada".
- **Social-Emotional:** Shows preferences, exhibits stranger anxiety.

Individual Variability

- Development varies widely among babies. Focus on progression rather than exact timing. Regular pediatric visits support monitoring and early intervention if needed.

Common Health Concerns: Symptoms and When to Seek Help

During the first year of life, babies can be prone to a variety of health issues, ranging from mild to severe. This guide helps you identify common concerns, recognize symptoms, and understand when to seek medical advice, ensuring you're prepared to manage your baby's health effectively. The aim is to empower parents with the knowledge and confidence to address their baby's health needs effectively.

Diaper Rash

- **Symptoms:** Redness and soreness in the diaper area.
- **Action:** Change diapers frequently, allow air drying, use barrier creams. Seek medical advice if the rash is severe, persistent, or accompanied by blisters.

Common Colds

- **Symptoms:** Runny/stuffy nose, cough, mild fever.
- **When to Seek Help:** If the baby has trouble breathing, refuses to feed, or has a fever (especially under 3 months old).

Fever Management

- **Important:** Any fever in a baby under 3 months is a medical emergency. In older babies, fever with lethargy, rash, or difficulty breathing requires a doctor's visit.

Allergies and Intolerances

- **Symptoms:** Hives, eczema, vomiting, diarrhea, fussiness.
- **Action:** Consult a pediatrician for suspected allergies/intolerances. Dietary adjustments or allergist evaluation may be necessary.

Serious Conditions

- **Alerts:** Persistent vomiting/diarrhea, unusual lethargy, difficulty breathing, signs of seizures.
- **Immediate Action:** Such symptoms demand prompt medical attention due to their potential severity.

Supporting Your Baby's Development: Activities and Play

Engaging in activities and play is essential for your baby's cognitive, physical, and emotional development. Activities and play are pivotal for a baby's development, offering opportunities for cognitive, physical, and emotional growth. This guide suggests age-appropriate play ideas to support developmental milestones, fostering a stimulating environment for your baby.

Newborns (0-3 Months)

- **Activities:** Engage in sensory play like gentle touch, soft music, and showing high-contrast images. Encourage early social interaction through soft talking and gentle cuddling.
- **Objective:** Stimulate senses and promote early social skills.

Infants (3-6 Months)

- **Interactive Play:** Incorporate tummy time with colorful toys and mirrors to build neck and upper body strength. Play peek-a-boo for social development and offer toys with various textures for tactile exploration.
- **Goals:** Enhance alertness, response to surroundings, and physical development.

Older Infants (6-12 Months)

- **Movement and Exploration:** Create safe spaces for crawling and walking practice. Use toys like blocks and shape sorters to improve fine motor skills and problem-solving. Support language development through singing, reading, and simple word use.
- **Focus:** Encourage mobility, fine motor skills, and language acquisition.

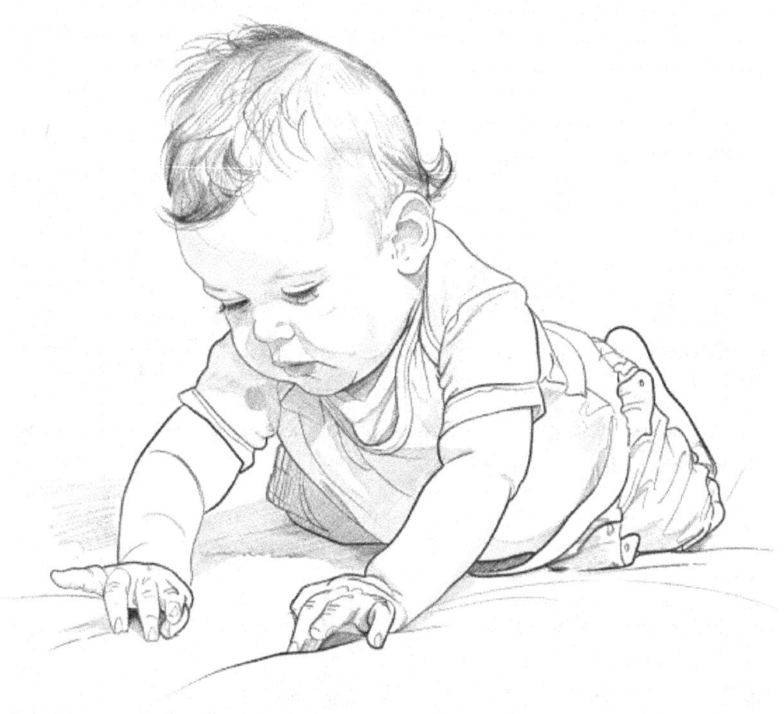

Crawling

Promoting Bonding Through Play

- The interaction during play, such as making eye contact and engaging in verbal and non-verbal communication, is key to bonding and enhances the play's developmental benefits.

Safety First

- Ensure toys and activities are safe and age-appropriate, supervising playtime to prevent accidents.

7

Your Health and Well-being

Main Idea: Overall, this chapter aims to underscore the importance of holistic care for new mothers, recognizing that their health and well-being are paramount for both their own recovery and their ability to nurture their newborns. Through practical advice and compassionate insight, this chapter seeks to support mothers in navigating the complexities of the postpartum period with confidence and care.

Physical Recovery After Birth: What to Expect

Postpartum recovery is a critical time as your body heals from childbirth and returns to its per-pregnancy state. This guide outlines expected physical changes and offers advice on managing common postpartum symptoms, emphasizing patience and self-care.

Healing and Symptoms Post-Childbirth

- **Vaginal Soreness and Lochia:** Expect vaginal soreness and bleeding (lochia) for several weeks.
- **Care for Tears/Incisions:** For vaginal deliveries, manage any perineal tears or episiotomy incisions with cleanliness and recommended care. After a cesarean section, follow specific care instructions for the incision site to aid healing and prevent infection.
- **Recovery Timeline:** Recovery varies, with the initial intensive period often lasting 6-8 weeks. Prioritize rest and gradually reintroduce

activities based on your healing progress and healthcare provider's advice.

Common Postpartum Symptoms

- **Fatigue, Mood Changes, and Discomfort:** Fatigue and mood fluctuations are common. Physical discomforts might include breast engorgement and uterine contractions as the uterus shrinks back.
- **Management Strategies:** Rest, nutrition, hydration, and approved pain relief methods are vital for managing these symptoms.

When to Seek Medical Attention

- **Warning Signs:** Fever, severe pain, infection signs at incision or episiotomy sites, and heavy bleeding or large clots require immediate medical consultation.

Nutrition and Fitness: Getting Back to Your Pr-Pregnancy Self

Regaining strength and fitness postpartum is vital for a new mother's health and well-being. This guide provides practical advice on nutrition and exercise, emphasizing realistic goals and listening to your body.

Nutrition for Postpartum Recovery and Breastfeeding

- **Balanced Diet:** Prioritize a diet rich in fruits, vegetables, lean proteins, whole grains, and healthy fats. Essential nutrients, including iron, calcium, vitamin D, and omega-3, are crucial for recovery and breastfeeding.
- **Hydration:** Essential for milk production, aim for adequate daily water intake.

Reintroducing Exercise

- **Listen to Your Body:** Consult with a healthcare provider before starting any postpartum exercise. Begin with gentle activities like walking and pelvic floor exercises, gradually increasing intensity.
- **Realistic Goals:** Set achievable fitness goals. Opt for shorter, manageable workouts that fit your new routine, and celebrate progress.

Balancing Motherhood and Fitness

- **Integrate Baby into Workouts:** Incorporate your baby into activities, such as stroller walks or baby-nearby yoga, to balance motherhood and fitness.
- **Support Networks:** Leverage support from family, friends, or postpartum exercise groups for motivation and accountability.

Emotional Well-being: Coping with Postpartum Mood Disorders

Postpartum recovery involves significant emotional adjustments. This guide addresses the spectrum of postpartum emotions, from the "baby blues" to more severe mood disorders like postpartum depression (PPD) and anxiety, offering guidance on identifying symptoms, coping strategies, and the importance of seeking professional help.

Understanding the Spectrum

- **Baby Blues:** Characterized by mood swings, sadness, and anxiety, appearing a few days post-birth and typically resolving within two weeks.
- **Postpartum Depression and Anxiety:** More severe and persistent symptoms include prolonged sadness, excessive worry, difficulty bonding with the baby, appetite or sleep changes, and thoughts of self-harm or harming the baby.

Effective Coping Strategies

- **Self-care:** Emphasize rest, balanced diet, physical activity, and personal relaxation time.
- **Social Support:** Lean on partners, family, and friends for support and connect with fellow new mothers for shared experiences and empathy.

Seeking Professional Help

- **Vital Step:** Consulting a healthcare provider for symptoms of PPD or anxiety is crucial. Treatment options may include therapy, support groups, or medication.
- **Early Intervention:** Key to rapid recovery and minimizing the impact on mother and child.

Finding Support: Building Your Parenting Community

No new mother should have to navigate the postpartum period in isolation. Creating a support network is crucial for receiving emotional backing, sharing experiences, and getting practical help. This guide highlights ways to connect and form a community that supports new mothers through the early stages of parenthood.

Leveraging Family and Friends

- **Open Communication:** Clearly express your needs for household help, meal prep, or company to your immediate circle. Loved ones often want to assist but might need direction on how to be most helpful.

Engaging with Parenting Groups

- **Join Groups:** Participate in local or online parenting groups for support and advice. These communities offer a chance to connect with peers in similar situations, sharing tips and experiences.

Healthcare Providers as a Resource

- **Professional Support:** Utilize pediatricians, obstetricians, and mental health experts for advice and referrals to resources like support groups and counseling, specifically geared towards new mothers.

Partner Communication

- **Collaborate with Partners:** Keep an open dialogue with your partner about mutual support. Sharing childcare duties, managing expectations, and allocating personal time can enhance your partnership during this transition.

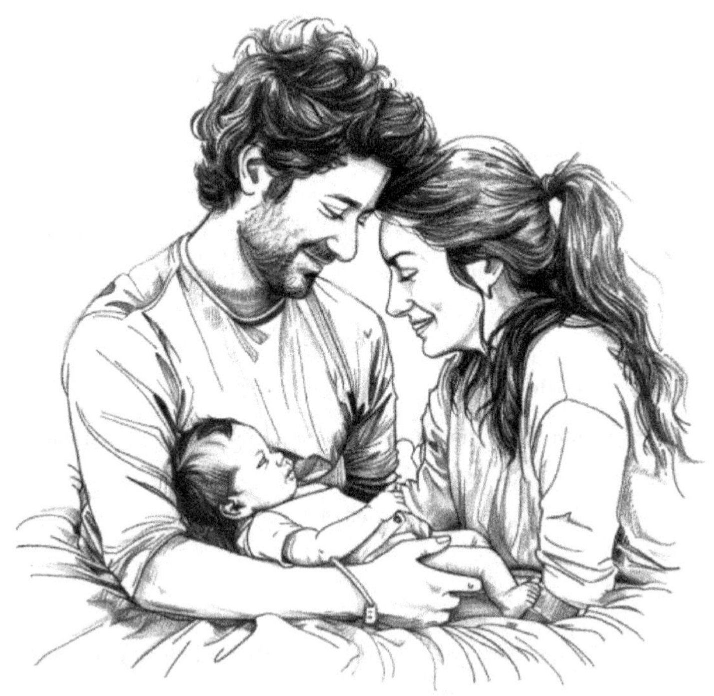

Bonding & mutual support

Online Forums and Social Media

- **Digital Communities:** Take advantage of online forums and social media for round-the-clock advice and connection, offering interaction with a global network of parents.

8

Balancing Work and Parenthood

Main **Idea:** This chapter aims to equip working parents with the tools and knowledge needed to navigate the complexities of balancing professional life with the responsibilities and joys of parenthood. By planning your return to work, selecting suitable childcare, managing your time effectively, and staying connected with your baby, you can create a fulfilling life that encompasses both your career aspirations and your family commitments.

Planning Your Return to Work: Maternity Leave and Beyond

Transitioning back to work after the arrival of a baby is a major shift that necessitates thorough preparation. This guide outlines essential steps for a seamless re-entry into the workforce post-maternity leave, focusing on effective communication with employers, the exploration of flexible work options, and managing the emotional journey of balancing career and new parental duties.

Communicating with Your Employer

- **Early Discussions:** Initiate conversations about your return date and flexibility needs well ahead of time. This openness allows for mutual preparation, potentially exploring part-time hours, remote work opportunities, or a phased return to full-time status.

Exploring Flexible Work Options

- **Flexible Arrangements:** Modern workplaces may offer flextime, telecommuting, job sharing, or compressed workweeks. Propose how such arrangements can benefit your productivity and job satisfaction as part of your plan to balance work and family life.

Emotional Preparation

- **Addressing Feelings:** The return to work can stir guilt, anxiety, and worry about childcare. Discussing these feelings with partners or support networks and practicing separation with trial childcare runs can ease this transition emotionally for both parent and child.

Managing Guilt and Anxiety

- **Positive Focus:** Combat guilt by concentrating on the benefits of working, such as professional fulfillment and financial stability for your family. Emphasize the importance of setting a strong work ethic example for your child and prioritize quality family time to maintain a close bond.

Childcare Options: Finding the Best Fit for Your Family

Finding suitable childcare is pivotal for working parents, impacting family dynamics, your child's development, and daily logistics. This guide delves into the variety of childcare options, highlighting the advantages and considerations of each to aid in making an informed decision that resonates with your family's preferences and requirements.

Daycare Centers:

- **Overview:** Daycare centers provide structured, group care focusing on education and social interaction.
- **Considerations:** Evaluate staff-to-child ratios, facility safety, educational philosophy, operational hours, and accreditation status to gauge quality and fit.

In-Home Nannies:

- **Overview:** Personalized care in your home, offering tailored support and flexibility.
- **Key Factors:** Assess experience, qualifications, compatibility with your parenting philosophy, reliability, and conduct thorough interviews and reference checks. A trial period can also be beneficial.

Family Care:

- **Advantages:** Care by known, trusted family members aligning with your values.
- **Communication is Key:** Discuss expectations, schedules, and any compensation clearly to avoid misunderstandings and ensure mutual satisfaction.

Vetting Providers and Making a Choice:

- **Due Diligence:** Regardless of childcare type, thoroughly vetting providers is essential. Visit facilities or meet caregivers, inquire about their discipline approach, emergency handling, daily routines, and observe interactions with your child to judge comfort and care quality.

Questions to Ask:

- What is your childcare experience and background?
- How do you communicate with parents about daily activities and child development?
- Can you provide references?
- What is your policy on sick days and vaccinations?
- Describe a typical day or activities planned.

Work-Life Balance: Tips for Managing Your Time

- Balancing work and family life is crucial for parents, particularly when adapting to parenthood. This section offers strategies to efficiently manage your time, ensuring you fulfill professional duties while enjoying family life. The focus is on practical organization, self-care, and quality family interactions to foster a balanced lifestyle.

Setting Clear Priorities

- **Assess and prioritize your tasks:** based on current family and professional needs. Focusing on what truly matters helps direct your energy effectively, enhancing both family well-being and career progress.

Utilizing Technology

- **Embrace technology:** to simplify tasks and organize schedules. Apps for time management, grocery delivery, and family calendars can save time for family interactions. Remote work and flexible hours can also aid in harmonizing work and family obligations.

Setting Boundaries

- **Define and maintain clear boundaries:** between work and home. Designate work hours and ensure family time is uninterrupted. Communicate these boundaries to colleagues and family to manage expectations.

Self-Care is Essential

- **Prioritize self-care** as a fundamental aspect of your routine, vital for your well-being and ability to care for others. Engage in activities that rejuvenate you, improving stress management and happiness.

Quality Over Quantity

- **Focus on the quality of time** spent with family. Be fully present during family activities, turning everyday moments into opportunities for connection and bonding.

Integrate Work and Family Life

- **Merge work and family life:** where possible, involving your family in work-related discussions and finding activities that reflect your professional interests. This integration can enhance mutual understanding and appreciation.

Staying Connected: Bonding with Your Baby Amidst a Busy Schedule

- Balancing work and parenting is challenging, yet maintaining a strong bond with your baby is crucial for their development and your relationship. This section provides strategies for busy parents to ensure meaningful connections with their baby, emphasizing the importance of quality time and engagement.

Maximizing Quality Time

- Use every opportunity, including playtime, feeding, and daily care routines, to interact positively with your baby. These moments, filled with attention and affection, reinforce your bond.

Establishing Routines

- Create consistent daily routines like morning activities, mealtimes, and bedtime rituals. Consistency offers a sense of security for your baby and sets aside dedicated times for bonding.

Incorporating Your Baby into Daily Activities

- Involve your baby in your everyday tasks. Using a baby carrier or placing them in a bouncer nearby allows them to be part of your day, promoting closeness even during mundane activities.

Using Technology to Stay Connected

- For parents away from home, technology can bridge the gap. Share pictures, videos, or have video calls to maintain a visual and emotional connection with your baby throughout the day.

Being Fully Present

- Focus entirely on your baby during bonding times. Minimize distractions to ensure these moments are engaging and meaningful, enhancing the emotional connection.

Self-Compassion and Patience

- Acknowledge the challenge of balancing work and family. Remember, small efforts in bonding are significant, and being patient with yourself is essential for sustainable parenting.

9

The Growing Family

Main **Idea:** This chapter aims to support families as they navigate the journey of growth and change, providing practical advice and emotional support for the challenges and joys of welcoming new members. By planning thoughtfully for siblings, actively maintaining and nurturing relationships, and adapting to the evolving family dynamics, parents can create a loving, supportive environment that fosters strong bonds and individual growth for all family members.

Deciding on More Children: Timing and Considerations

Expanding your family with more children is a significant decision impacting everyone involved. This section explores the timing, how to discuss a new sibling with your current children, and preparing them for becoming older siblings, aiming for a well-rounded approach that considers the whole family's well-being.

Timing Considerations

Choosing when to add to your family involves several factors: the age gap between siblings, parental ages, career implications, and overall family lifestyle. Smaller gaps might foster close sibling bonds, while larger gaps can give parents more one-on-one time with each child and give older siblings a sense of independence.

Discussing with Existing Children

When introducing the idea of a new sibling, it's crucial to involve your current children in the discussion, highlighting the positive aspects and addressing any concerns. This conversation should reassure them of your unchanging love and attention.

Preparing for the Role of Older Sibling(s)

Preparing your child for an older sibling role goes beyond conversations. Include them in pregnancy-related activities, like setting up the nursery, to build excitement and a feeling of responsibility. Reading books about getting a new sibling and emphasizing their important role can also be beneficial.

Family Dynamics

Consider how a new addition will affect family dynamics, including daily routines, attention distribution, and financial resources. A new baby changes family life, and it's vital to ensure your family is ready to embrace these changes positively.

Making an Informed Decision

The decision to have more children should consider emotional, logistical, and financial aspects. Open discussions with your partner about your feelings, concerns, and expectations are essential, as is seeking advice from those who've faced similar decisions or professional guidance.

Sibling Dynamics: Preparing Your First Child

When welcoming a new baby into the family, it's crucial to prepare your first child for the changes ahead to minimize feelings of jealousy and ensure they feel included and important. This section outlines practical steps to help your first child adapt to their new role and foster a loving relationship with the new sibling.

Involving Your Child in the Pregnancy

Involve your first child in the pregnancy process to help them feel connected to the new sibling. This can include sharing the news in an exciting way, involving them in nursery preparations, and inviting them to prenatal appointments if possible. Such involvement helps build anticipation and a sense of responsibility.

Setting Expectations

Discuss what having a new baby means, focusing on both the demands and the joys of a sibling. It's essential to convey that while the baby will need a lot of care, the love within the family will grow. Ensure your first child knows they play a unique and valued role in the family.

Addressing Feelings of Jealousy

Talk openly about any worries or jealousy your first child may feel towards the new baby. Validate their feelings and reassure them of your love and attention. Keeping their routine consistent can also provide a sense of security.

Facilitating Sibling Bonding

Encourage interactions between your first child and the new baby under your supervision. Involve them in age-appropriate caregiving tasks and praise them for gentle behavior, reinforcing the bond between siblings.

Modeling Positive Sibling Relationships

Show positive interactions between siblings through your actions and stories. Read books about becoming a big brother or sister to help them understand and get excited about their new role.

Keeping the Spark Alive: Nurturing Your Relationship

Introducing new members to the family, while enriching, also puts new demands on the parental relationship. It's essential for parents to actively nurture their bond, ensuring the family's foundation remains strong and loving despite these pressures. This section provides actionable strategies for couples to stay connected and support each other through the journey of parenting.

Prioritizing the Relationship

Acknowledge the importance of your partnership as the foundation of your family. Make a conscious effort to set aside quality time together, whether it's for date nights, shared activities, or quiet moments amidst the chaos of family life.

Open Communication

Maintain open lines of communication, discussing needs, feelings, and daily experiences freely. This helps prevent misunderstandings and builds mutual empathy and understanding, keeping the relationship strong.

Maintaining Intimacy

Intimacy can be challenged by parenting demands. Strive to keep the emotional and physical connection alive through affection, spending quality time together, and expressing love and appreciation for each other.

Sharing Responsibilities

Share parenting and household duties to alleviate stress and foster teamwork. Fairly dividing tasks and acknowledging each other's efforts can strengthen your sense of partnership.

Finding Time for Each Other

In the hustle of family life, finding time for each other might require planning. Consider arranging childcare for date nights, setting aside time for daily check-ins, or finding moments to connect throughout the day.

Facing Challenges Together

Tackle parenting and family challenges as a team. Approach problems with a mindset focused on solutions and mutual support, strengthening your bond through each obstacle and celebration.

Family Planning: Financial and Emotional Preparedness

Expanding your family involves significant emotional and financial preparation. This section provides a detailed guide for parents considering more children, covering how to financially and emotionally prepare for this life-changing decision.

Financial Planning and Budgeting

Understanding the financial implications of adding to your family is critical. Assess your finances, including savings, expenses, and income. Create a budget that accounts for additional costs such as healthcare, childcare, education, and daily necessities. Look for ways to boost income or cut back on non-essential expenses to accommodate the new financial demands.

Establishing a Financial Safety Net

An emergency fund becomes even more crucial when expanding your family. Aim to save enough to cover several months' expenses for unforeseen financial challenges. Review and adjust your insurance policies—health, life, and disability—to ensure they adequately cover your growing family's needs.

Emotional Readiness and Support Systems

The emotional aspect of adding a new family member is equally important. Consider your family's emotional capacity to welcome another child and the impact on current dynamics. Discuss with your partner and children their feelings about a new family member, ensuring everyone's emotions and thoughts are acknowledged.

Strengthening Support Networks

A robust support network is invaluable. This includes family, friends, and community resources that can offer both emotional and practical support. Identify how these networks can assist you, from childcare to emotional support, and strengthen these connections in anticipation of your family's growth.

Preparing Siblings for a New Arrival

If you have other children, prepare them for their new role as older siblings. Involve them in preparations for the new arrival and discuss their feelings and expectations, reinforcing their importance in the family and addressing any concerns they may have.

Prioritizing Self-Care

Parental self-care is vital during this transition. The demands of expanding your family can strain your emotional and physical well-being. Maintain open communication with your partner about your needs and invest in self-care practices. Seek professional support if necessary to navigate this period healthily.

10

Looking Ahead: Beyond the First Year

Main Idea: This chapter aims to guide parents through the toddler years and beyond, providing a foundation of knowledge and strategies for navigating the complexities of raising a growing child.

By focusing on development, parenting styles, continuous learning, and the power of celebration and traditions, this chapter equips parents to foster a nurturing, supportive, and joyful family life.

As your baby transitions from infancy to toddler hood, the journey of parenting shifts to new challenges, milestones, and opportunities for growth—for both the child and the parents.

This chapter is designed to provide insight into the developmental stages that follow the baby's first year, exploring toddler development, the exploration of parenting styles, the importance of continuing education for parents, and ways to celebrate milestones and create lasting family traditions.

Through this guidance, parents can navigate the coming years with confidence, equipped with the knowledge to support their child's growth and foster a nurturing family environment.

Toddler Milestones: Physical and Emotional Development

As your baby transitions into the toddler years, expect a whirlwind of development, from physical abilities like walking and talking to emotional growth such as feeling expression and empathy building. This phase is also when independence starts to shine, with milestones like self-feeding and the early stages of toilet training coming into play.

Walking and Motor Skills

By the toddler years, most children begin to walk unaided, with their mobility rapidly advancing to running, climbing, and jumping. Encourage these physical skills by providing a safe, open space for exploration and play. Activities like kicking a ball or building with blocks can further refine their motor skills and hand-eye coordination.

Language and Communication

Language development takes off during this period. Support their burgeoning vocabulary by engaging in conversations, reading together, and naming objects and emotions during daily routines. Singing songs and reciting nursery rhymes also boost language acquisition.

Self-Feeding and Early Toilet Training

Toddlers start showing interest in self-feeding with utensils and may begin to show readiness for toilet training. Introduce self-feeding in a mess-friendly environment and look for signs of toilet training readiness, such as staying dry for longer periods or showing interest in the bathroom, introducing the concept gradually and positively.

Emotional Development and Social Skills

Emotionally, toddlers learn to express a range of feelings and start developing empathy. They may also start forming early friendships. Encourage emotional intelligence by talking about feelings, modeling empathy, and facilitating playdates or group activities to nurture social skills.

Encouraging Independence Safely

While promoting independence, it's crucial to ensure safety. Childproof your home to prevent accidents and provide a secure environment for your toddler to explore and learn. Balancing supervision with the freedom to explore is key to fostering their independence and confidence.

Fostering Curiosity and Learning

Toddlers are naturally curious. Stimulate their learning by providing a variety of age-appropriate toys and activities that challenge and engage them. Regular outings, interactive play, and new experiences can also support their cognitive development and curiosity about the world.

Parenting Styles: Finding What Works for Your Family

During the toddler years, choosing a parenting style that aligns with your family's values and meets your child's individual needs becomes particularly important. This section discusses the four main parenting styles—authoritative, authoritarian, permissive, and uninvolved—and examines their effects on child behavior and development.

Authoritative Parenting: This style combines warmth and structure, offering children clear guidelines and expectations while also encouraging independence and providing emotional support. Authoritative parents use positive discipline strategies, promote open communication, and value mutual respect. Studies suggest this approach leads to children who are confident, self-reliant, and socially adept.

Authoritarian Parenting: Authoritarian parents enforce strict rules and expect obedience without question. Communication is more one-sided, and there's less emphasis on nurturing the child's emotional needs. While this style can lead to compliance, it may also foster lower self-esteem and increased anxiety or aggression in children.

Permissive Parenting: Permissive parents are indulgent and lenient, often setting few boundaries and allowing children significant freedom. While these parents are typically loving and communicative, the lack of structure can lead to difficulties with self-discipline and frustration in situations where rules and cooperation are necessary.

Uninvolved Parenting: Uninvolved parenting is characterized by a lack of responsiveness to a child's needs. Minimal communication, limited supervision, and negligible affection are common. This approach can result in significant emotional and behavioral issues, with children often struggling with self-esteem and academic achievement.

Continuing Education: Resources for Ongoing Learning

The journey of parenting doesn't stand still; as your child grows, the challenges and opportunities for parental growth evolve as well. This section highlights the importance of ongoing learning for parents, pointing you towards a variety of resources designed to keep you informed and effective in your parenting role.

Books: There is a wealth of books covering every imaginable parenting topic, from toddler nutrition and sleep strategies to managing behavior and understanding developmental milestones. Regularly seeking out new publications can keep you up-to-date with the latest research and advice.

Workshops and Seminars: Many communities offer workshops and seminars on parenting topics. These sessions not only provide valuable information but also offer the chance to ask questions and interact with experts in the field.

Online Courses: The internet is a treasure trove of online courses and webinars tailored to parents. Covering broad themes or focusing on niche subjects, these courses allow you to learn at your own pace and on your own schedule.

Groups: Joining a parenting support group, whether in-person or online, can provide you with a network of peers facing similar challenges. These groups offer emotional support, practical advice, and the opportunity to share experiences and strategies.

Parenting Blogs and Websites: Digital platforms offer a continuous stream of articles, blogs, and forums where parents can find tips, support, and community. From expert-led sites to personal blogs, the diversity of perspectives can be both enlightening and reassuring.

Social Media and Podcasts: Social media networks and parenting podcasts can be excellent sources of quick tips, deep dives into specific topics, and stories from other parents. They're ideal for busy parents looking for accessible, on-the-go advice.

Celebrating Milestones: Making Memories and Traditions

Marking milestones and creating family traditions are vital for building a strong family identity and fostering joy. This part outlines ways to celebrate key moments like birthdays, developmental achievements, and cultural or religious holidays, offering suggestions for crafting memorable traditions that resonate with your family's unique values and heritage.

Birthdays and Achievements: Beyond the usual birthday party, consider personalized rituals that can become eagerly anticipated annual events, such as a special outing, a unique gift that ties into an interest or a milestone, or a family activity that reflects the birthday person's preferences. For achievements, create a tradition of celebratory dinners where the focus is on the accomplishment, encouraging storytelling and expressions of pride.

Cultural and Religious Holidays: Use these occasions to deepen your child's understanding of and connection to their cultural or religious heritage. This might involve traditional meals, storytelling, participating in community events, or creating specific family activities that highlight the holiday's significance.

Seasonal Traditions: Each season offers opportunities for unique family traditions. From the first day of spring picnics, summer beach days, autumn leaf collecting, to winter snow walks, these activities can become cherished annual events that your child looks forward to.

Creating Memories: Documenting these milestones and traditions through photos, videos, or a family journal can create a treasure trove of memories for your child to look back on. Consider creating a digital archive or a physical scrapbook that can be added to over the years.

Involving Your Child: As your child grows, involve them in choosing, planning, and evolving family traditions. This inclusion not only makes celebrations more meaningful to them but also teaches them about decision-making and the importance of family bonds.

Flexibility and Simplicity: While traditions are important, they should not become a source of stress. It's okay for traditions to evolve or be simplified as your family's needs and circumstances change. The essence of these traditions lies in the togetherness they foster, not in their complexity or execution.

11

Conclusion

In wrapping up this guide, we reflect on the comprehensive journey of parenting, from the anticipation of pregnancy to the transformative experience of childbirth and navigating the crucial early years of your child's life. This book has aimed to arm you with essential knowledge and practical advice for the various stages of early parenthood, providing a foundation for confident and informed parenting decisions.

Parenting is a dynamic journey of growth, discovery, and deep love, punctuated by both challenges and victories. As you progress, it's vital to trust in your inherent capabilities as a parent, supported by the knowledge that your dedication forms the bedrock of your child's future.

The importance of seeking support cannot be overstated. Parenting is a shared experience, enriched by the wisdom and encouragement of a broader community including family, friends, healthcare professionals, and fellow parents.

This collective support system is invaluable, offering guidance and companionship through the ups and downs of raising children.

Take time to cherish every moment with your child. The early years, while sometimes challenging, are filled with milestones that are fleeting and precious. Embrace these times, as they are the building blocks of lifelong memories and joy.

As this book concludes, we encourage you to share your own journey, contributing your unique experiences to the wider narrative of parenthood. Your insights can offer invaluable support to others on a similar path. We invite you to leave a review on Amazon, sharing how this guide has impacted your parenting journey, thus enriching the broader dialogue on the challenges and rewards of raising children.

Thank you for inviting us into your parenting journey. May this book remain a valuable resource as you continue to navigate the wondrous path of raising your child. Here's to the journey ahead—filled with learning, love, and the immeasurable joy of family.

12

References

Books

1. American Academy of Pediatrics. (2018). *AAP Schedule of Well-Child Care Visits*. Retrieved from https://www.aap.org/en-us/Pages/Default.aspx

2. Centers for Disease Control and Prevention. (2020). *Recommended Vaccinations for Infants and Children (Birth through 6 Years)*. Retrieved from https://www.cdc.gov/vaccines/schedules/hcp/imz/child-adolescent.html

3. Dewar, G. (2019). *Parenting Science – The Science of Child-Rearing and Child Development*. Retrieved from https://www.parentingscience.com

4. Gonzalez, A., & James, C. (2017). *The Motherhood Manual: Strategies and Tips for the First Year*. New York, NY: Parenting Press.

5. Hogg, T., & Blau, M. (2005). *Secrets of the Baby Whisperer for Toddlers*. New York, NY: Ballantine Books.

6. Karp, H. (2015). *The Happiest Baby on the Block: Fully revised and updated second edition. The New Way to Calm Crying and Help Your Newborn Baby Sleep Longer*. New York, NY: Bantam Books.

7. Murkoff, H., & Mazel, S. (2016). *What to Expect the First Year*. New York, NY: Workman Publishing Company.

8. Oster, E. (2019). *Cribsheet: A Data-Driven Guide to Better, More Relaxed Parenting, from Birth to Preschool*. New York, NY: Penguin Press.

9. Siegel, D.J., & Payne Bryson, T. (2012). *The Whole-Brain Child: 12 Revolutionary Strategies to Nurture Your Child's Developing Mind*. New York, NY: Delacorte Press.

10. World Health Organization. (2020). *Infant and Young Child Feeding*. Retrieved from https://www.who.int/nutrition/topics/infantfeeding/en/

11. American Academy of Pediatrics. (2021). *Caring for Your Baby and Young Child: Birth to Age 5* (7th ed.). Bantam. A comprehensive guide covering health, behavioral, and developmental issues from infancy through preschool.

12. Centers for Disease Control and Prevention. (2021). *Early Childhood Nutrition*. Retrieved from https://www.cdc.gov/nutrition/infantandtoddlernutrition/index.html. Guidelines on providing proper nutrition for infants and toddlers to support healthy growth.

13. Duncan, G. J., & Magnuson, K. (2013). Investing in preschool programs. *Journal of Economic Perspectives, 27*(2), 109-132. A study on the benefits of early childhood education programs on long-term developmental outcomes.

14. Ginsburg, K. R. (2007). *The Importance of Play in Promoting Healthy Child Development and Maintaining Strong Parent-Child Bonds*. American Academy of Pediatrics. Analysis of how play contributes to children's physical and emotional well-being.

15. Harvard University Center on the Developing Child. (2020). *Key Concepts: Brain Architecture*. Retrieved from https://developingchild.harvard.edu/science/key-concepts/brain-architecture/. An overview of how early experiences affect the development of the brain.

16. Lieberman, A. F., & Van Horn, P. (2008). *Psychotherapy with Infants and Young Children: Repairing the Effects of Stress and Trauma on Early Attachment*. The Guilford Press. This book delves into therapeutic approaches for addressing early trauma in young children.

17. National Institute of Child Health and Human Development. (2017). *Safe to Sleep® Public Education Campaign*. Retrieved from https://safetosleep.nichd.nih.gov/. Guidelines and research findings on reducing the risk of sudden infant death syndrome (SIDS).

18. Shonkoff, J. P., & Phillips, D. A. (Eds.). (2000). *From Neurons to Neighborhoods: The Science of Early Childhood Development*.

National Academies Press. An extensive examination of early childhood development and the influences of environment and care.

19. Siegel, D. J. (2020). *Mind: A Journey to the Heart of Being Human*. W. W. Norton & Company. Explores the neuroscience of human experience, with implications for parenting and child development.

20. Zero to Three. (2021). *Baby Brain Map*. Retrieved from https://www.zerotothree.org/resources/529-baby-brain-map. Interactive tool explaining infant brain development and its impact on early learning.

21. Brazelton, T. B., & Sparrow, J. (2008). *Touchpoints-Three to six*. Da Capo Lifelong Books.

22. Ginsburg, K. R., & Jablow, M. M. (2014). *Building resilience in children and teens: Giving Kids Roots and Wings*.

23. Leach, P. (2022). *Your baby and child: From Birth to Age Five*. Dorling Kindersley Ltd.

24. Siegel, D. J., & Hartzell, M. (2023). *Parenting from the Inside Out: How a Deeper Self-understanding Can Help You Raise Children who Thrive*.

25. Gottman, J., PhD, & Gottman, J. S., PhD. (2008). *And baby makes three: The Six-Step Plan for Preserving Marital Intimacy and Rekindling Romance After Baby Arrives*. Harmony.

Medical Websites

1. *Infant and young child feeding: Model Chapter for textbooks for medical students and allied health professionals*. (2009).

2. Cook, W. J., & Klaas, K. M. (2020). *Mayo Clinic Guide to your baby's first years: Newborn to Age 3*. Rosetta Books.

3. Pediatrics, A. a. O. (2017). *Bright futures: Guidelines for Health Supervision of Infants, Children, and Adolescents*.

4. Offit, P. A., & Bell, L. M. (2003). *Vaccines: What You Should Know*. John Wiley & Sons.

5. Dowshen, S., Izenberg, N., & Bass, E. (2002). *The KidsHealth Guide for Parents*. McGraw Hill Professional.

6. *HealthyChildren.org - from the American Academy of Pediatrics*. (n.d.). HealthyChildren.org. https://www.healthychildren.org/

Research Studies and Journals

1. Ainsworth, M. D. S., Blehar, M. C., Waters, E., & Wall, S. N. (2015). *Patterns of attachment: A Psychological Study of the Strange Situation*. Psychology Press.

2. Bowlby, J. (1988). Developmental psychiatry comes of age. *American Journal of Psychiatry*, *145*(1), 1–10. https://doi.org/10.1176/ajp.145.1.1

3. Bowlby, J. (1997). *Attachment and Loss: Attachment*. Random House.

4. Varga, L. (2022). On the Bridge between Paediatric Neurology and Early Childhood Pedagogy. In *University of Sopron Press eBooks* (pp. 5–20). https://doi.org/10.35511/978-963-334-425-5-varga

5. Weatherston, D. J. (2001). Infant Mental health. *Psychoanalytic Social Work*, *8*(1), 43–74. https://doi.org/10.1300/j032v08n01_04

Additional Resources

- ZERO TO THREE. (2024, February 7). *ZERO TO THREE | Early connections last a lifetime*. https://www.zerotothree.org/

- Staff, P. T. (2022, January 24). *Home*. Child Development Institute. https://childdevelopmentinfo.com/